The RAD (Rare Adipose Disorder) Diet for Lipedema

A Beginner's 3-Week Step-by-Step Plan with Recipes & a 7-Day Meal Guide to Manage Symptoms

copyright © 2025 Isadora Kwon

All rights reserved No part of this book may be reproduced, or stored in a retrieval system, or transmitted in any form or by any means, electronic, mechanical, photocopying, recording, or otherwise, without express written permission of the publisher.

Disclaimer

By reading this disclaimer, you are accepting the terms of the disclaimer in full. If you disagree with this disclaimer, please do not read the guide.

All of the content within this guide is provided for informational and educational purposes only, and should not be accepted as independent medical or other professional advice. The author is not a doctor, physician, nurse, mental health provider, or registered nutritionist/dietician. Therefore, using and reading this guide does not establish any form of a physician-patient relationship.

Always consult with a physician or another qualified health provider with any issues or questions you might have regarding any sort of medical condition. Do not ever disregard any qualified professional medical advice or delay seeking that advice because of anything you have read in this guide. The information in this guide is not intended to be any sort of medical advice and should not be used in lieu of any medical advice by a licensed and qualified medical professional.

The information in this guide has been compiled from a variety of known sources. However, the author cannot attest to or guarantee the accuracy of each source and thus should not be held liable for any errors or omissions.

You acknowledge that the publisher of this guide will not be held liable for any loss or damage of any kind incurred as a result of this guide or the reliance on any information provided within this guide. You acknowledge and agree that you assume all risk and responsibility for any action you undertake in response to the information in this guide.

Using this guide does not guarantee any particular result (e.g., weight loss or a cure). By reading this guide, you acknowledge that there are no guarantees to any specific outcome or results you can expect.

All product names, diet plans, or names used in this guide are for identification purposes only and are the property of their respective owners. The use of these names does not imply endorsement. All other trademarks cited herein are the property of their respective owners.

Where applicable, this guide is not intended to be a substitute for the original work of this diet plan and is, at most, a supplement to the original work for this diet plan and never a direct substitute. This guide is a personal expression of the facts of that diet plan.

Where applicable, persons shown in the cover images are stock photography models and the publisher has obtained the rights to use the images through license agreements with third-party stock image companies.

Table of Contents

Introduction 7
Taking Control of Lipedema Through Nutrition 9
   How Diet Affects Lipedema: The Science Behind the RAD Approach ... 11
   The Role of the RAD Diet 13
What Is the RAD (Rare Adipose Disorder) Diet? 15
   The Principles of Eating for Lipedema Management ... 16
   Key Nutrients to Focus On: Anti-Inflammatory & Lymphatic Support Foods ... 17
   Foods to Eat and Avoid for Lipedema ... 20
Meal Planning & Grocery Shopping for Success 23
   Creating a Lipedema-Friendly Grocery List ... 23
   How to Read Food Labels to Avoid Triggers ... 26
   Budget-Friendly Shopping Tips for Clean Eating ... 28
   Kitchen Staples & Easy Meal Prep Hacks ... 31
Recipes for Lipedema Management 35
   Breakfast: Anti-Inflammatory & Metabolism-Boosting Options ... 36
   Berry Chia Pudding ... 37
   Veggie-Packed Breakfast Scramble ... 38
   Green Smoothie Bowl ... 39
   Sweet Potato & Avocado Breakfast Bowl ... 40
   Cinnamon Almond Butter Overnight Oats ... 41
   Lunch: Light, Nutrient-Dense, and Filling Meals ... 42
   Mediterranean Quinoa Salad ... 43
   Turkey Lettuce Wraps ... 44
   Creamy Zucchini Soup ... 45
   Rainbow Veggie Grain Bowl ... 46
   Lentil Veggie Wraps ... 47
   Dinner: Protein-Rich & Balanced Recipes for Symptom Control ... 48
   Herb-Crusted Salmon with Steamed Vegetables ... 49
   Zoodles with Turkey Meatballs ... 50
   Coconut Chicken Stir-Fry ... 51

    Garlic Herb Chicken with Cauliflower Mash   52
    Shrimp and Spinach Stir-Fry   53
    Snacks & Drinks: Hydration and Healthy Fat-Focused Options   54
    Avocado Dip with Veggie Sticks   55
    Hydrating Lemon-Ginger Tea   56
    Coconut Energy Bites   57
    Spiced Pumpkin Seed Mix   58
    Cooling Cucumber-Mint Infused Water   59

The 7-Day Lipedema Meal Plan   **60**
    How to Use This Meal Plan for Maximum Results   60
    Sample Weekly Menu Breakdown   61
    Portion Sizes & Adjustments for Your Needs   65
    Meal Prepping for a Smooth Week Ahead   66

The 3-Week RAD Diet Action Plan   **68**
    Week 1: Reset & Eliminate Triggers   68
    Week 2: Nourish & Replenish   75
    Week 3: Long-Term Sustainability   82

Lifestyle Habits to Support Lipedema Management   **90**
    The Role of Movement: Gentle Exercises to Improve Circulation   90
    Managing Stress & Reducing Inflammation Holistically   92
    Sleep, Recovery, and Self-Care Practices for Lipedema   93
    Supplements: Do You Need Them?   94
    How to Maintain the RAD Diet Long-Term   96
    Common Pitfalls & How to Overcome Them   97
    Additional Resources & Support Groups   98

Conclusion   **100**
FAQs   **102**
References and Helpful Links   **105**

Introduction

Lipedema is a complex condition characterized by an abnormal buildup of fat in specific areas of the body, often leading to disproportionate swelling, tenderness, and mobility challenges. Misunderstanding surrounding the condition can lead to frustration and delayed care as it's frequently mistaken for obesity or other medical concerns. Managing its symptoms requires a comprehensive approach that addresses the root contributors to discomfort, such as inflammation, poor circulation, and fluid retention.

The RAD Diet, short for Rare Adipose Disorder Diet, has been specifically developed to meet the unique needs of those managing lipedema. This nutrition plan moves beyond traditional weight-loss diets by targeting the triggers that worsen lipedema symptoms.

It emphasizes healing through nutrient-dense foods that promote anti-inflammatory responses, support a healthy lymphatic system, and stabilize blood sugar levels. Carefully selecting foods, like leafy greens, omega-3 fatty acid-rich sources, and low-glycemic carbohydrates, helps reduce symptom severity while nourishing the body.

Combined with lifestyle changes, the RAD Diet aims to create a manageable pathway toward improved well-being. Gentle exercise, such as walking or swimming, contributes to improved circulation and lymphatic flow. Practices like stress management and self-care complement dietary habits, enhancing the effectiveness of symptom management and promoting long-term health.

In this guide, we will talk about the following:

- Taking Control of Lipedema Through Nutrition
- What is the RAD (Rare Adipose) Diet?
- Meal Planning & Grocery Shopping for Success
- Recipes for Lipedema Management
- The 7-Day Lipedema Meal Plan
- The 3-Week RAD Diet Action Plan
- Lifestyle Habits to Support Lipedema Management

Keep reading to learn more about the RAD Diet and how it can help improve your quality of life while managing lipedema symptoms. By the end , you will have a better understanding of how proper nutrition and lifestyle changes can make a significant impact on your health and well-being.

Taking Control of Lipedema Through Nutrition

Lipedema is a chronic disorder of fat metabolism that most commonly affects women. It causes an abnormal buildup of fat cells, typically in the lower body, such as the hips, thighs, legs, and sometimes arms, which can make those areas look disproportionately larger compared to the rest of the body. This condition can often be mistaken for obesity, lymphedema, or other weight-related concerns, but it is a distinct condition with unique challenges.

Key Characteristics of Lipedema

1. *Symmetrical Fat Distribution*: Lipedema fat buildup typically happens equally on both sides of the body. For example, both legs may appear larger, while the upper body remains unaffected or less affected.
2. *Painful to the Touch*: Unlike regular fat, the areas affected by lipedema are often tender or painful when touched or with slight pressure.

3. ***Bruising & Fragility***: Many people with lipedema notice easy bruising in affected areas due to weakened capillaries and poor circulation.
4. ***Diet-Resistant Fat***: A hallmark of lipedema is that the excess fat does not respond well to traditional weight-loss methods, such as calorie restriction or increased exercise.

The Daily Challenges of Lipedema

Living with lipedema can be physically, emotionally, and socially challenging. Some of the key hurdles include:

- ***Mobility Issues***: Swollen and heavy legs can make it difficult to walk long distances or engage in physical activities.
- ***Chronic Discomfort or Pain***: The heaviness and tenderness often lead to long-term physical discomfort.
- ***Self-Esteem Concerns***: Many people with lipedema struggle with body image issues, judgment from others, or lack of awareness about their condition.
- ***Poor Circulation***: Swelling and lymphatic system impairment lead to fluid retention, which worsens the overall symptoms.

Left unmanaged, lipedema can progress and increase the risk of complications, including lymphedema (swelling caused by lymph fluid buildup). Managing this condition requires a holistic approach, and one of the most important aspects of that is nutrition.

How Diet Affects Lipedema: The Science Behind the RAD Approach

Diet plays a critical role in managing lipedema because the food we eat directly impacts inflammation, lymphatic function, and overall metabolic health. While there is no universal "cure" for lipedema, a conscious approach to diet can help manage symptoms, slow progression, and improve quality of life.

The Connection Between Lipedema & Nutrition

1. **Inflammation**

    Chronic inflammation is a core issue in lipedema. Foods that trigger inflammation in the body—such as refined sugars, artificial additives, and processed foods—can exacerbate swelling, tenderness, and fluid retention. On the other hand, anti-inflammatory foods, like leafy greens, fatty fish, and spices such as turmeric, may help soothe inflammation.

2. **Lymphatic System Support**

    The lymphatic system is vital for removing waste and toxins from the body. However, in lipedema, lymph flow is often compromised, which worsens swelling and fat accumulation. A well-balanced diet that encourages hydration and provides lymphatic-supportive nutrients (like potassium, magnesium, and antioxidants) can promote better lymph flow. For example, cucumbers, celery, and herbal teas are natural lymphatic boosters.

3. **Blood Sugar Control & Insulin Sensitivity**

   People with lipedema may experience worsened symptoms if their diet causes spikes in blood sugar and insulin levels. High-sugar and high-carbohydrate foods can lead to fat storage in the body, which may amplify the buildup of lipedema fat. By focusing on low-glycemic foods like legumes, nuts, and non-starchy vegetables, you help stabilize blood sugar and reduce fat-triggering mechanisms.

4. **Fluid Retention**

   Lipedema leads to fluid buildup in affected areas, which causes swelling and heaviness. Foods that are high in salt or sodium contribute to water retention, making the symptoms worse. Switching to minimally processed foods and increasing potassium-rich options, like avocados and bananas, can help balance fluid levels in the body.

By making mindful dietary changes, individuals with lipedema can reduce inflammation, support lymphatic function, and manage symptoms like swelling and fluid retention. Prioritizing a balanced, nutrient-rich diet can play a key role in improving overall quality of life.

The Role of the RAD Diet

The RAD Diet (Rare Adipose Disorder Diet) does more than just eliminate harmful foods—it actively introduces healing nutrients that work to minimize lipedema symptoms. Here's what the RAD Diet focuses on and why it's effective:

- *Anti-Inflammatory Foods*: By emphasizing foods high in omega-3 fatty acids (like salmon or walnuts) and vitamins (such as antioxidants in berries), the RAD Diet helps fight chronic inflammation—a major driver of pain and swelling in lipedema.
- *Hydration & Electrolytes*: Drinking enough water and incorporating foods that support hydration (like cucumbers and watermelon) boost lymphatic flow and reduce fluid retention.
- *Nutrient Density*: A lipedema-focused diet avoids "empty calories" and focuses on meals packed with vitamins, minerals, protein, and healthy fats to energize and support healing.

Why Dietary Changes Work in Lipedema Management

The symptoms of lipedema may feel daunting, but diet gives people a tangible way to regain control of their health. Reducing inflammatory triggers, improving lymphatic health, and balancing blood sugar all contribute to a drastic reduction in swelling, pain, and discomfort.

Through the RAD Diet, we can reframe "dieting" from something restrictive to something empowering, where each meal is an opportunity to give your body the tools it needs to thrive. The RAD Diet emphasizes sustainable, everyday changes to avoid "diet fatigue." It's not about what you can't eat; it's about discovering what foods work with your body, not against it.

When paired with other strategies like exercise, stress reduction, and self-care, the RAD Diet becomes an essential part of a well-rounded plan to live better with lipedema.

Both understanding the condition and making intentional food choices can feel overwhelming at first, but this guide will break it all down into actionable steps in the coming chapters. Together, we'll focus on foods you can love that also help you feel your best, one meal at a time.

What Is the RAD (Rare Adipose Disorder) Diet?

The RAD Diet, short for Rare Adipose Disorder Diet, is a nutrition plan specifically tailored to address the unique challenges of managing lipedema. Unlike traditional diets that often focus solely on weight loss, the RAD Diet recognizes the complexities of lipedema as a condition impacted by inflammation, lymphatic health, and structural fat retention.

Instead of targeting general calorie deficits, the RAD Diet emphasizes healing the body by choosing nutrient-dense, whole foods that alleviate lipedema symptoms, reduce swelling, and support overall well-being.

The RAD Diet empowers those with lipedema to focus on what they can control through intentional eating habits. It's not about deprivation or one-size-fits-all solutions. Instead, it's about using food as a tool to reduce inflammation, nourish the lymphatic system, and promote long-term health. You're not just eating to survive; you're eating to thrive.

The Principles of Eating for Lipedema Management

A successful RAD Diet centers around several key principles that align with the unique needs of those managing lipedema. These principles shift the focus away from weight loss gimmicks and instead prioritize symptom control and overall health.

1. *Focus on Whole, Unprocessed Foods*: Foods in their natural state provide essential nutrients to fight inflammation and support physical health. This includes fresh vegetables, fruits, lean proteins, and healthy fats.
2. *Eliminate Common Food Triggers*: Inflammatory foods like processed sugars, refined carbs, artificial additives, and trans fats can exacerbate swelling and discomfort. Avoiding these is essential for maintaining balance in the body.
3. *Adopt an Anti-Inflammatory Eating Style*: Prioritize meals featuring leafy greens, fatty fish, berries, nuts, and spices like turmeric. These foods have properties that actively fight inflammation and soothe discomfort.
4. *Support Your Lymphatic System*: Lipedema negatively affects lymphatic circulation, leading to fluid retention and swelling. Staying hydrated and eating foods that help flush fluid, such as cucumber, celery, and citrus fruits, is vital.

5. ***Create a Balance of Macronutrients***: Every meal should focus on a balance of protein, healthy fats, and low-glycemic carbohydrates. Together, these can stabilize blood sugar levels, reduce fat-promoting insulin spikes, and keep energy levels steady throughout the day.
6. ***Prioritize Sustainability Over Perfection***: The RAD Diet is intended to be adaptable. It's not about perfection or strict rules; it's about finding what works for your symptoms and preferences. Small, consistent changes can make a big impact over time.

By focusing on nourishing, anti-inflammatory foods and supporting your lymphatic system, the RAD Diet offers a sustainable approach to managing lipedema symptoms. Small, consistent changes can lead to improved health and greater comfort over time.

Key Nutrients to Focus On: Anti-Inflammatory & Lymphatic Support Foods

Eating for lipedema requires paying close attention to specific nutrients that promote healing and alleviate symptoms like swelling, pain, and fatigue. These nutrients have been carefully chosen to address the root causes of lipedema symptoms.

1. ***Omega-3 Fatty Acids***: Omega-3s reduce inflammation in the body, helping to ease pain and discomfort caused by swollen areas. These healthy fats also support heart health, which can be impacted when dealing with lipedema.

   <u>Best Sources:</u>
   - Salmon
   - mackerel
   - walnuts
   - chia seeds
   - Flaxseeds

2. ***Antioxidants***: Antioxidants fight damage caused by free radicals, reduce oxidative stress, and soothe inflammation. These are especially beneficial for reducing chronic pain and supporting skin health.

   <u>Best Sources:</u>
   - Blueberries
   - spinach
   - kale
   - raspberries
   - red bell peppers

3. ***Potassium & Magnesium***: These minerals are essential for reducing water retention and supporting lymphatic circulation. They also aid in muscle relaxation and reduce cramping.

Best Sources:

- Avocados
- bananas
- leafy greens
- almonds
- sunflower seeds

4. ***Protein***: Protein is necessary for repairing tissues, supporting muscle strength, and balancing blood sugar levels. It also helps with feelings of fullness, reducing unnecessary snacking

Best Sources:

- Grass-fed meats
- eggs
- wild-caught fish
- lentils
- tofu

5. ***Hydrating Foods***: Proper hydration promotes lymphatic drainage and reduces swelling. Foods rich in water content and electrolytes are perfect for encouraging fluid balance.

Best Sources:

- Cucumber
- celery
- watermelon
- citrus fruits

- bone broth

Foods to Eat and Avoid for Lipedema

Choosing the right foods isn't just about following a list — it's about understanding how those foods work with your body's unique chemistry to alleviate symptoms and support better health. While every individual may have specific tolerances or preferences, the following guidelines are a solid starting point.

Foods to Eat

Focus on a variety of nutrient-rich, whole foods that offer anti-inflammatory and lymphatic-support benefits.

- *Proteins*: Chicken breast, turkey, salmon, grass-fed beef, eggs, tofu, lentils, and beans.
- *Vegetables*: Spinach, kale, zucchini, broccoli, cauliflower, carrots, cucumbers, asparagus, and bell peppers.
- *Fruits*: Blueberries, strawberries, avocados, oranges, grapefruits, cherries, and apples (in moderation).
- *Healthy Fats*: Avocado, olive oil, coconut oil, nuts (like almonds and walnuts), seeds (like flax and chia).
- *Whole Grains & Low-Glycemic Carbs*: Quinoa, chickpeas, black beans, sweet potatoes, and oats (complex carbs help maintain energy and avoid insulin spikes).

- ***Drinks***: Herbal teas (like dandelion or nettle), water with lemon or cucumber, and bone broth.

Incorporating these nutrient-dense, anti-inflammatory foods into your diet can support overall health and promote optimal body function. Focus on balance and variety to nourish your body and maintain energy levels throughout the day.

Foods to Avoid

Certain foods can add stress to your body by triggering inflammation, water retention, or blood sugar spikes.

- ***Refined Sugars***: Sodas, candies, baked goods, and other processed sweets.
- ***Processed Foods***: Packaged snacks, frozen ready meals, and fast food.
- ***Trans Fats & Hydrogenated Oils***: Found in many margarines, fried foods, and processed snacks.
- ***High-Sodium Foods***: Canned soups, deli meats, salty chips, and overly seasoned sauces.
- ***Gluten (for some people)***: Many individuals with lipedema note reduced swelling and bloating when avoiding gluten.
- ***Alcohol***: Can trigger inflammation and promote water retention, making symptoms worse for many.

Avoiding certain foods can help reduce inflammation, water retention, and other stressors in your body. By making mindful dietary choices, you can better manage symptoms and support your overall well-being.

Meal Planning & Grocery Shopping for Success

Meal planning and grocery shopping are essential steps in successfully managing lipedema through the RAD Diet. With the right strategies, you'll build a foundation to consistently choose foods that alleviate symptoms while keeping things easy, affordable, and enjoyable.

Creating a Lipedema-Friendly Grocery List

Building a grocery list tailored to lipedema management is a key step in staying on track with the RAD Diet. Here's how to create a list that supports your health and simplifies your shopping experience.

Essential Categories to Include:

1. *Proteins*: Focus on anti-inflammatory, high-quality protein sources to repair tissues and maintain muscle strength.

    <u>Examples:</u>
    - Organic Chicken

- turkey
- wild-caught fish
- eggs
- lentils
- tofu
- grass-fed beef

2. ***Vegetables***: Choose fresh, colorful, and nutrient-dense veggies to support your lymphatic system and reduce inflammation.

   Examples:

   - Spinach
   - kale
   - zucchini
   - cucumbers
   - broccoli
   - bell peppers
   - celery
   - Asparagus

3. ***Fruits***: Opt for low-sugar, antioxidant-rich fruits to stabilize blood sugar and combat oxidative stress.

   Examples:

   - Blueberries
   - raspberries
   - avocados
   - cherries

- citrus fruits

4. ***Healthy Fats***: Include fats that reduce inflammation and provide sustained energy.

   Examples:

   - Avocado
   - olive oil
   - coconut oil
   - nuts (almonds, walnuts)
   - seeds (chia, flax)

5. ***Low-Glycemic Carbs***: Add slow-digesting carbs that won't spike insulin levels.

   Examples:

   - Sweet potatoes
   - quinoa
   - chickpeas
   - Oats

6. ***Hydrating Foods***: Support lymphatic drainage with foods high in water content.

   Examples:

   - Watermelon
   - cucumber
   - celery
   - citrus fruits

Tips for Building Your List:

- Plan meals for the week ahead and base your list on recipes or meal ideas.
- Stick to the outer aisles of the grocery store, where fresh, whole foods are typically found.
- Keep pantry staples like spices, oils, and dry goods stocked to make meal prep easier.

By organizing your grocery list into these categories, you'll make healthier choices and set yourself up for success with the RAD Diet.

How to Read Food Labels to Avoid Triggers

Understanding food labels is essential for managing lipedema. Many processed foods contain hidden ingredients that can worsen inflammation, fluid retention, and other symptoms. Here's how to decode labels and make informed choices.

Key Things to Look For:

1. **Ingredient List:**
    - Choose products with short, simple ingredient lists made up of whole, recognizable foods.
    - Avoid items with long lists of chemicals or additives you can't pronounce.

2. **Added Sugars:**
   - Watch for hidden sugars, which can appear under names like "syrup," "sucrose," "fructose," or "maltodextrin."
   - Aim for products with little to no added sugar.
3. **Sodium Content:**
   - High sodium levels can lead to water retention, and worsening swelling.
   - Look for items with 140 mg of sodium or less per serving.
4. **Trans Fats and Oils:**

   Avoid products with "hydrogenated" or "partially hydrogenated" oils, as these are trans fats that promote inflammation.

5. **Serving Size:**

   Pay attention to serving sizes to ensure you're not consuming more sugar, sodium, or calories than intended.

Common Triggers to Avoid:

- *Processed Sugars*: Found in candies, baked goods, and sugary drinks.
- *Gluten (if sensitive)*: Some people with lipedema find gluten worsens symptoms.

- ***Artificial Additives***: Preservatives, flavor enhancers (like MSG), and artificial colors can trigger inflammation.
- ***High-Sodium Packaged Foods***: Processed snacks, canned soups, and frozen meals often contain excessive salt.

Quick Tips for Smarter Choices:

- Opt for whole, unprocessed foods whenever possible.
- Choose "low sodium," "unsweetened," or "no added sugar" options.
- Be cautious of "health" claims like "low-fat" or "sugar-free," as these often contain hidden additives.

By mastering food labels, you'll avoid common dietary triggers and make choices that support your lipedema management goals.

Budget-Friendly Shopping Tips for Clean Eating

Eating clean and managing lipedema doesn't have to break the bank. With a few smart strategies, you can enjoy nutrient-rich, anti-inflammatory foods while staying within your budget.

1. **Shop Seasonally and Locally**
   - **Why it works**: Seasonal produce is often cheaper, fresher, and more flavorful. Local

farmers' markets or co-ops can offer great deals on fresh fruits and vegetables.
- **Pro tip**: Look for "ugly" or imperfect produce, which is just as nutritious but often sold at a discount.

2. **Buy in Bulk**
   - **Why it works**: Staples like quinoa, lentils, oats, nuts, and seeds are more affordable when purchased in larger quantities.
   - **Pro tip:** Check the bulk aisle or warehouse stores for deals on pantry essentials. Store them in airtight containers to keep them fresh.

3. **Choose Frozen Over Fresh (When Needed)**
   - **Why it works:** Frozen fruits and vegetables are often less expensive and last longer. They're picked at peak ripeness, so they retain their nutrients.
   - **Pro tip:** Stock up on frozen spinach, berries, and broccoli for quick, healthy meal options.

4. **Meal Prep to Minimize Waste**
   - **Why it works:** Planning meals in advance helps you buy only what you need, reducing food waste and saving money.
   - **Pro tip:** Use leftovers creatively—turn roasted veggies into soups or salads, and repurpose proteins like chicken into wraps or stir-fries.

5. **Prioritize Basics Over Gourmet Items**
   - **Why it works:** Whole, unprocessed foods like vegetables, grains, and proteins are often cheaper and more nutritious than trendy "health" products.
   - **Pro tip:** Skip pre-packaged "clean eating" snacks and make your own, like roasted chickpeas or homemade trail mix.
6. **Stick to a List**
   - **Why it works:** A well-planned grocery list helps you avoid impulse buys and stick to your budget.
   - **Pro tip:** Plan meals for the week and shop with a list based on your recipes.
7. **Use Store Brands**
   - **Why it works:** Many store-brand products are just as good as name brands but cost significantly less.
   - **Pro tip:** Compare labels to ensure the quality and ingredients match your needs.
8. **Cook at Home**
   - **Why it works:** Preparing meals at home is far cheaper than eating out or buying pre-made meals.
   - **Pro tip:** Batch cook soups, stews, and casseroles to freeze for future meals.

By following these tips, you can enjoy clean, lipedema-friendly eating without overspending. A little planning goes a long way in making healthy eating both affordable and sustainable!

Kitchen Staples & Easy Meal Prep Hacks

Setting up your kitchen for lipedema management is all about having the right tools at your fingertips. Stocking up on essential staples and learning a few meal prep tricks can make sticking to the RAD Diet simple and stress-free. Here's how to create a lipedema-friendly kitchen that supports your health and saves you time.

Essential Kitchen Staples

1. **Pantry Staples:** These long-lasting items are the backbone of many lipedema-friendly meals, providing nutrients and ease of preparation.
    - *Whole Grains & Legumes*: Quinoa, lentils, chickpeas, black beans, rolled oats.
    - *Healthy Oils*: Extra virgin olive oil, avocado oil, coconut oil.
    - *Nuts & Seeds*: Almonds, walnuts, sunflower seeds, chia seeds, flaxseeds.
    - *Spices & Seasonings*: Turmeric, paprika, garlic powder, onion powder, cinnamon, ginger.
    - *Low-Sodium Options*: Low-sodium broth, canned organic beans (rinsed before use).

- *Non-Dairy Milk*: Unsweetened almond, coconut, or cashew milk.
2. **Fridge Staples:** Keep your fridge stocked with fresh, nutrient-rich foods to build quick and healthy meals.
    - *Proteins*: Eggs, organic chicken or turkey, wild-caught fish, tofu.
    - *Fresh Vegetables*: Spinach, kale, zucchini, cucumbers, broccoli, bell peppers.
    - *Hydration Essentials*: Citrus fruits, celery, watermelon, cucumbers.
    - *Fermented Foods*: Sauerkraut, kimchi, or yogurt (unsweetened, non-dairy options like almond or coconut yogurt).
3. **Freezer Staples:** Frozen items are a lifesaver for time-pressed days and help reduce food waste.
    - *Vegetables*: Broccoli, spinach, cauliflower rice, mixed veggie blends.
    - *Fruits*: Blueberries, raspberries, mango chunks, bananas (peeled and sliced for smoothies).
    - *Proteins*: Pre-cooked chicken, wild-caught salmon fillets, veggie burgers.
    - *Bone Broth*: Perfect for soups or hydrating meals.

By having these staples on hand, you'll always have the building blocks for nutritious, lipedema-friendly meals.

Easy Meal Prep Hacks

1. **Batch Cooking:**
   - Cook a large quantity of quinoa, lentils, or roasted veggies early in the week. Divide into portions to use in salads, wraps, or bowls.
   - Bake or grill chicken breasts or fish fillets in bulk, then freeze for future meals.

2. **Pre-Chopping Ingredients:**
   - Chop veggies like onions, bell peppers, and zucchini and store them in airtight containers in the fridge.
   - This makes it easy to toss them into soups, stir-fries, or omelets.

3. **Invest in Storage Solutions:**
   - Use glass containers to portion out meals for the week. Label them for quick grab-and-go lunches or dinners.
   - Store nuts, seeds, and grains in airtight jars for easy access and prolonged freshness.

4. **Make Base Ingredients Multitask:**
   - Roast sweet potatoes or carrots and use them as a side dish, a salad topping, or blended into soups.
   - Bone broth can be used as the base for soups or enjoyed on its own as a snack.

5. **Prepare Grab-and-Go Snacks:**

- Pre-measure nuts, seeds, and fresh fruit into snack bags or containers.
- Make chia pudding or overnight oats in mason jars for a quick breakfast option.

6. **One-Pot and Sheet Pan Meals:**
    - Use one pan to roast chicken, sweet potatoes, and veggies for a complete meal with minimal cleanup.
    - Create soups or stews in a slow cooker for an easy, savory meal packed with nutrients.

7. **Smoothie Freezer Packs:**

Prep smoothie ingredients (frozen fruit, spinach, chia seeds) into bags and freeze. Simply toss into the blender with non-dairy milk when needed.

8. **Keep a Weekly Menu Plan:**
    - Plan meals in advance and designate specific days for certain staples (e.g., "Grain Bowl Mondays" or "Soup Sundays").
    - This reduces decision fatigue and keeps your diet varied yet structured.

By combining these meal prep hacks with a well-stocked kitchen, you'll save time, stay on budget, and make healthy choices easier—giving you a strong foundation for managing lipedema through the RAD Diet.

Recipes for Lipedema Management

Eating for lipedema doesn't mean depriving yourself of delicious meals. With the RAD Diet as your foundation, it's easy to create flavorful dishes that support your health. This chapter includes practical recipes and tips for every meal of the day, helping you reduce inflammation, manage symptoms, and feel satisfied.

Breakfast: Anti-Inflammatory & Metabolism-Boosting Options

Fuel your day with breakfasts packed with anti-inflammatory ingredients and metabolism-friendly nutrients.

Berry Chia Pudding

Ingredients:

- 3 tbsp chia seeds
- 1 cup unsweetened almond milk
- 1/2 tsp pure vanilla extract
- 1/2 cup fresh or frozen blueberries
- 1/4 cup walnuts (optional)

Instructions:

1. Combine chia seeds, almond milk, and vanilla in a jar or bowl. Stir well.
2. Refrigerate overnight, stirring once after 1 hour to prevent clumping.
3. Top with blueberries and walnuts before serving.

Veggie-Packed Breakfast Scramble

Ingredients:

- 2 eggs or egg whites
- 1/2 cup spinach (chopped)
- 1/4 cup diced red bell pepper
- 1/4 cup zucchini (chopped)
- 1 tsp olive oil
- Salt and pepper to taste

Instructions:

1. Heat olive oil in a skillet over medium heat.
2. Add bell peppers and zucchini, cooking until tender.
3. Add spinach and stir for 1 minute until wilted.
4. Whisk eggs in a bowl, then pour into the skillet. Cook and scramble to mix with veggies. Season with salt and pepper.

Green Smoothie Bowl

Ingredients:

- 1 frozen banana
- 1/2 avocado
- 1 cup spinach
- 1 tbsp chia seeds
- 1/2 cup unsweetened coconut milk
- Toppings: shredded coconut, blueberries, pumpkin seeds

Instructions:

1. Blend all ingredients until smooth.
2. Pour into a bowl and add desired toppings.

Sweet Potato & Avocado Breakfast Bowl

Ingredients:

- 1 small sweet potato (baked and mashed)
- 1/2 avocado (sliced)
- 1 tbsp chia seeds
- 1 boiled egg (optional)
- Sprinkle of sea salt and paprika

Instructions:

1. Bake or microwave the sweet potato until soft, then mash it.
2. Add avocado slices, a boiled egg (if desired), and chia seeds.
3. Sprinkle with salt and paprika for additional flavor.

Cinnamon Almond Butter Overnight Oats

Ingredients:

- 1/2 cup rolled oats
- 1 cup unsweetened almond milk
- 1 tbsp almond butter
- 1/2 tsp cinnamon
- 1 tsp chia seeds

Instructions:

1. Mix all ingredients in a jar or container. Stir well.
2. Refrigerate overnight. Serve cold or warm up in the microwave the next morning.

Lunch: Light, Nutrient-Dense, and Filling Meals

These lunches are light, easy to prepare, and packed with nutrients to sustain you through the afternoon.

Mediterranean Quinoa Salad

Ingredients:

- 1 cup cooked quinoa
- 1/2 cup cucumber (diced)
- 1/4 cup cherry tomatoes (halved)
- 2 tbsp red onion (finely chopped)
- 2 tbsp olive oil
- Juice of 1 lemon
- 1/4 cup crumbled feta cheese (optional)
- Salt and pepper to taste

Instructions:

1. In a bowl, mix together quinoa, cucumber, cherry tomatoes, and red onion.
2. Combine lemon juice and olive oil, then pour it over the salad.
3. Toss well, add salt and pepper, and top with feta if desired.

Turkey Lettuce Wraps

Ingredients:

- 4 large lettuce leaves (e.g., butterhead or romaine)
- 4 oz cooked turkey breast or ground turkey
- 1/4 avocado (sliced)
- 1/4 cup shredded carrots
- 1 tbsp hummus

Instructions:

1. Arrange lettuce leaves on a plate. Spread a thin layer of hummus on each.
2. Fill with turkey, carrots, and avocado slices. Wrap them up and enjoy.

Creamy Zucchini Soup

Ingredients:

- 2 medium zucchinis (chopped)
- 1 small onion (chopped)
- 2 cups low-sodium vegetable broth
- 1 tbsp olive oil
- 1/4 cup coconut milk
- Salt and pepper to taste

Instructions:

1. Heat olive oil in a pot, and cook onion until translucent.
2. Add zucchini and broth. Bring to a boil, then simmer for 10–12 minutes.
3. Blend the mixture until smooth, stir in coconut milk, and season to taste.

Rainbow Veggie Grain Bowl

Ingredients:

- 1/2 cup cooked quinoa or brown rice
- 1/4 cup shredded purple cabbage
- 1/4 cup shredded carrots
- 1/4 cup diced cucumber
- 1/4 avocado (sliced)
- 2 tbsp tahini dressing

Instructions:

1. Layer the quinoa or rice in a bowl. Top with cabbage, carrots, cucumber, and avocado slices.
2. Drizzle with tahini dressing before serving.

Lentil Veggie Wraps

Ingredients:

- 1/2 cup cooked lentils
- 1 whole-grain or gluten-free wrap
- 1/4 cup shredded lettuce
- 1/4 cup diced tomatoes
- 1 tbsp hummus

Instructions:

1. Spread hummus onto the wrap.
2. Layer with lentils, lettuce, and tomatoes. Fold and roll into a wrap.

Dinner: Protein-Rich & Balanced Recipes for Symptom Control

Evening meals should include ample protein, healthy fats, and minimal carbohydrates to support symptom control.

Herb-Crusted Salmon with Steamed Vegetables

Ingredients:

- 1 salmon fillet (5–6 oz)
- 1 tbsp olive oil
- 1 tsp dried dill
- 1 tsp garlic powder
- 1 cup steamed broccoli and carrots

Instructions:

1. Preheat oven to 375°F (190°C).
2. Coat salmon with olive oil, then sprinkle with dill and garlic powder.
3. Bake for 12–15 minutes. Serve with steamed vegetables.

Zoodles with Turkey Meatballs

Ingredients:

- 2 cups zucchini noodles (zoodles)
- 6 turkey meatballs (pre-cooked or homemade)
- 1/2 cup sugar-free marinara sauce
- 1 tbsp olive oil

Instructions:

1. Heat olive oil in a skillet, sauté zoodles for 2–3 minutes.
2. Heat meatballs and marinara sauce in a separate skillet.
3. Combine zoodles with sauce and meatballs. Serve warm.

Coconut Chicken Stir-Fry

Ingredients:

- 1 chicken breast (sliced into thin strips)
- 1 cup mixed bell peppers (sliced)
- 1/2 cup snap peas
- 2 tbsp coconut milk
- 1 tsp coconut oil
- 1 tsp ginger (grated)
- Salt and pepper to taste

Instructions:

1. Heat coconut oil in a skillet, and cook chicken strips until done. Remove and set aside.
2. Add bell peppers, snap peas, and ginger to the skillet. Stir-fry for 3–4 minutes.
3. Return chicken to the skillet, mix in coconut milk, and season with salt and pepper.

Garlic Herb Chicken with Cauliflower Mash

Ingredients:

- 2 chicken thighs (skinless)
- 1 tsp garlic powder
- 1 tsp dried rosemary or thyme
- 1 tbsp olive oil
- 1 cup cauliflower (steamed and mashed)

Instructions:

1. Preheat oven to 375°F (190°C). Season chicken thighs with garlic powder and rosemary.
2. Heat olive oil in an oven-safe skillet and sear the chicken for 2–3 minutes per side. Transfer the skillet to the oven and bake for 15 minutes.
3. Serve with mashed cauliflower seasoned with salt and pepper.

Shrimp and Spinach Stir-Fry

Ingredients:

- 1 cup shrimp (peeled and deveined)
- 2 cups fresh spinach leaves
- 1 tbsp coconut oil
- 1 tsp grated ginger
- 1 tsp coconut aminos (optional)

Instructions:

1. Heat coconut oil in a skillet over medium heat. Add shrimp and cook until pink, 3–4 minutes. Remove and set aside.
2. Add spinach and ginger to the skillet, stir-frying until wilted. Return shrimp to the pan and toss together. Flavor with coconut aminos if desired.

Snacks & Drinks: Hydration and Healthy Fat-Focused Options

Snacks are your chance to stay full and energized without overloading with sugar. Hydrating drinks can help with lymphatic drainage.

Avocado Dip with Veggie Sticks

Ingredients:

- 1 avocado (mashed)
- 1 tbsp lemon juice
- Salt and pepper to taste
- Veggie sticks (carrots, celery, bell peppers)

Instructions:

1. In a bowl, mix mashed avocado with lemon juice, salt, and pepper.
2. Serve with veggie sticks for dipping.

Hydrating Lemon-Ginger Tea

Ingredients:

- 1 cup hot water
- Juice of 1/2 lemon
- 1 tsp grated fresh ginger
- 1 tsp honey (optional)

Instructions:

1. Steep ginger in hot water for 5 minutes.
2. Add lemon juice and honey if desired.

Coconut Energy Bites

Ingredients:

- 1 cup almond flour
- 2 tbsp shredded coconut
- 2 tbsp coconut oil
- 1 tbsp chia seeds
- 1 tsp vanilla extract

Instructions:

1. Mix all ingredients in a bowl. Roll into small balls.
2. Refrigerate for 30 minutes before enjoying.

Spiced Pumpkin Seed Mix

Ingredients:

- 1/2 cup raw pumpkin seeds
- 1/2 tsp olive oil
- 1/4 tsp turmeric
- 1/4 tsp smoked paprika
- Pinch of sea salt

Instructions:

1. Preheat oven to 350°F (175°C). Toss pumpkin seeds with olive oil and spices in a bowl.
2. Spread onto a baking sheet and roast for 10–12 minutes. Cool before enjoying.

Cooling Cucumber-Mint Infused Water

Ingredients:

- 1/2 cucumber (sliced)
- 4–5 mint leaves
- 1 quart of filtered water

Instructions:

1. Combine cucumber slices and mint leaves in a jug of water.
2. Refrigerate for 2–4 hours to allow flavors to infuse.

With these recipes in your toolkit, you'll enjoy a delicious, nutrient-packed approach to lipedema management. Meal by meal, you'll feel more empowered and in control of your health!

The 7-Day Lipedema Meal Plan

Taking control of lipedema symptoms through food starts with a well-structured and manageable plan. The 7-Day Meal Plan is designed to help you transition seamlessly into the RAD Diet while reducing inflammation and boosting your energy. Use the meal plan as a roadmap to nourish your body and simplify your daily routine.

How to Use This Meal Plan for Maximum Results

Following the 7-Day Meal Plan is easy when you stay focused and organized. Here are steps to help you make the most of it:

1. ***Prep Ingredients in Advance:*** Set aside 1–2 hours at the start of the week to prepare staples like cooked quinoa, roasted veggies, grilled proteins, or smoothie packs. This saves time on busy weekdays.
2. ***Stick to Portion Sizes:*** Each meal is balanced to provide energy without overloading your system. Follow the recommended portions and avoid second servings.

3. ***Pair Meals with Hydration:*** Drink plenty of water and herbal teas. Mint- or cucumber-infused water is ideal to promote lymphatic drainage. Aim for at least 8 servings daily to stay hydrated.
4. ***Adjust for Your Needs:*** Feel free to swap meals or snacks within the same day or week. For example, you can have a leftover dinner for lunch to reduce cooking demand.
5. ***Incorporate Movement:*** Pair this plan with daily movements, like walking or gentle stretching. This helps manage fluid retention and inflammation.
6. ***Don't Stress About Perfection:*** If you slip up, don't worry—just get back to the plan with your next meal. It's about consistency, not perfection.

By following this plan with intention and flexibility, you'll set a solid foundation for symptom relief and overall well-being.

Sample Weekly Menu Breakdown

This sample menu includes breakfast, lunch, dinner, and snacks with specific recipes that follow RAD Diet principles. Adjust portions based on your individual needs.

Day 1

- ***Breakfast:*** Veggie-Packed Breakfast Scramble (spinach, bell peppers, eggs)
- ***Snack:*** Avocado Dip with Veggie Sticks (carrots and celery)

- *Lunch:* Mediterranean Quinoa Salad with olive oil and lemon dressing
- *Dinner:* Garlic Herb Chicken with Cauliflower Mash
- *Drink:* Lemon-Ginger Tea

Day 2

- *Breakfast:* Cinnamon Almond Butter Overnight Oats
- *Snack:* Pumpkin Seed Mix (roasted with turmeric and paprika)
- *Lunch:* Turkey Lettuce Wraps with hummus and shredded carrots
- *Dinner:* Shrimp and Spinach Stir-Fry with coconut aminos
- *Drink:* Cucumber-Mint Infused Water

Day 3

- *Breakfast:* Sweet Potato & Avocado Breakfast Bowl
- *Snack:* Coconut Energy Bites (almond flour, chia seeds, shredded coconut)
- *Lunch:* Rainbow Veggie Grain Bowl with tahini dressing
- *Dinner:* Zoodles with Turkey Meatballs and sugar-free marinara sauce
- *Drink:* Hydrating Lemon-Ginger Tea

Day 4

- *Breakfast:* Green Smoothie Bowl (banana, spinach, avocado, chia seeds)
- *Snack:* Fresh apple slices with almond butter
- *Lunch:* Lentil Veggie Wraps with gluten-free tortilla and hummus
- *Dinner:* Herb-Crusted Salmon with steamed broccoli and carrots
- *Drink:* Cucumber-Mint Infused Water

Day 5

- *Breakfast:* Berry Chia Pudding topped with walnuts and blueberries
- *Snack:* A boiled egg with a sprinkle of paprika
- *Lunch:* Creamy Zucchini Soup paired with a small green salad
- *Dinner:* Coconut Chicken Stir-Fry with snap peas and bell peppers
- *Drink:* Herbal tea with ginger and honey

Day 6

- *Breakfast:* Breakfast Scramble with zucchini and spinach
- *Snack:* Spiced Pumpkin Seed Mix for crunchy, on-the-go snacking
- *Lunch:* Leftover Herb-Crusted Salmon over leafy greens with olive oil

- **Dinner:** Garlic Herb Chicken and roasted sweet potatoes
- **Drink:** Unsweetened hibiscus tea for added hydration

Day 7

- **Breakfast:** Sweet Potato & Avocado Bowl with chia and a boiled egg
- **Snack:** A handful of raw almonds and sunflower seeds
- **Lunch:** Turkey Lettuce Wraps with avocado slices and shredded carrots
- **Dinner:** Shrimp Stir-Fry with roasted asparagus on the side
- **Drink:** Lemon-Ginger Tea

Tips for Success

1. ***Keep Your Kitchen Stocked***: Refer back to **Chapter 3** for pantry and freezer essentials to ensure you always have ingredients on hand.
2. ***Make It Fun***: Experiment with different spices, herbs, and garnishes to keep recipes interesting and enjoyable.
3. ***Track Your Progress***: Notice how these meals make you feel physically and emotionally, and make notes of your favorite dishes!

With this 7-day plan, you'll have a strong foundation to reduce inflammation and feel your best. Meal planning takes the guesswork out of eating for lipedema and gives you the tools to succeed in managing your symptoms.

Portion Sizes & Adjustments for Your Needs

Eating the right portion sizes is essential for symptom management and energy balance. Here are easy ways to determine and customize portions for your needs:

1. **Focus on the Plate Method**
    - Fill half your plate with non-starchy vegetables like leafy greens, zucchini, or peppers.
    - Use a quarter of your plate for lean protein like chicken, turkey, or lentils.
    - Reserve the final quarter for healthy fats like avocado, nuts, or seeds—or low-glycemic carbs like quinoa or sweet potatoes.
2. **Adjust for Activity Levels**
    - On high-energy days, add slightly larger portions of protein or carbs.
    - When you're less active, prioritize veggies and healthy fats to keep you full without adding unnecessary calories.
3. **Quick Visual References**
    - Protein (chicken, fish, or tofu): Palm-sized.
    - Fats (avocado, olive oil): Thumb-sized.
    - Carbs (quinoa, sweet potato): About ½ cup or your fist.

- Veggies (leafy greens, zucchini): Unlimited but avoid overloading with starchy ones.

By customizing portion sizes based on your activity level and using simple visual cues, you can maintain a balanced diet that supports your energy and health. Remember, small adjustments can make a big difference in managing symptoms and feeling your best.

Meal Prepping for a Smooth Week Ahead

Meal prepping simplifies your week and makes sticking to the RAD Diet stress-free. Here's how to plan and cook efficiently:

1. **Plan Your Menu First**: Review the weekly menu and shopping list before heading to the store. Buy ingredients in bulk to save time and money.
2. **Batch-Cook Staples**: Prepare large quantities of versatile items—quinoa, roasted veggies, grilled chicken, or stir-fry greens—that can be used in multiple meals.
3. **Store Meals & Ingredients Properly**: Use clear, airtight containers to portion out meals. Label each with the date to avoid food waste. Freeze extra portions of soups, stir-fries, or cooked grains for quick meals when you're busy.

4. ***Create Grab-and-Go Options***: Pre-cut veggies, portion snacks, and assemble smoothie packs in freezer bags to save time during busy mornings or mid-day cravings.
5. ***Maximize Flavor***: Keep olive oil, vinegar, herbs, and spices handy for quick seasoning. These add variety to your meals without extra prep time.
6. ***Schedule a Prep Day***: Designate a weekly "prep day" to cook, chop, and store ingredients. Spend 1–2 hours prepping to save hours during the week.

By prepping ahead, you'll eliminate guesswork, save time, and set yourself up for success every day of the week.

The 3-Week RAD Diet Action Plan

Taking control of your diet can feel like a big step, but by breaking it down into three manageable weeks, you can ease into lasting lifestyle changes. This 3-week RAD Diet Action Plan is designed to help you reset your system, nourish your body, and develop habits that will support you for the long term. You'll focus on simple, achievable goals each week, with specific daily guidance to keep you on track.

Week 1: Reset & Eliminate Triggers

This first week is all about starting fresh by removing inflammatory, processed, and artificial foods. Cleaning up your diet reduces swelling, stabilizes energy levels, and gives your body the reset it needs to perform its best. By the end of this week, you'll feel lighter, less bloated, and more in control of your health.

Goals for Week 1:

- ***Eliminate Processed Foods***: Say goodbye to packaged snacks, refined sugars, and junk foods that may trigger inflammation or slow your progress.

- *Focus on Nutrient-Dense Foods*: Build your meals using fresh vegetables, high-quality proteins, and healthy fats to fuel your body.
- *Hydrate Consistently*: Drinking enough water will help with lymphatic function and reduce puffiness or water retention.

This week might feel challenging at first if you're used to processed or packaged foods, but taking it one step at a time will make the transition manageable and rewarding.

Daily Breakdown for Week 1:

Day 1: Hydrate & Start Fresh

Starting your day with proper hydration sets the tone for a successful week. Water helps flush out toxins and supports your lymphatic system from the get-go.

Action Steps:

- First thing in the morning, drink a full glass of water. Add a squeeze of fresh lemon for a refreshing taste and an extra vitamin C boost.
- For meals, use fresh ingredients like grilled chicken, roasted vegetables, and avocado. These provide a balance of high-quality protein, vitamins, and healthy fats without unnecessary additives.

- Throughout the day, replace any sugary drinks like soda or juice with herbal teas or infused water (try adding cucumber or mint for flavor).

Example Recipe Idea:

Breakfast could be a simple two-egg vegetable scramble with spinach and tomatoes, paired with avocado slices and herbal tea.

Pro Tip: Invest in a reusable water bottle to track your daily water intake and make sure it's always accessible, whether you're at home or on the go.

Day 2: Cut Out Refined Carbs

Refined carbs such as white bread, pasta, and pastries are often hidden culprits that lead to inflammation and energy crashes. Swapping them out for healthier alternatives keeps meals satisfying without the negative effects.

Action Steps:

- Instead of bread or pasta, choose nutrient-rich substitutes like quinoa, sweet potatoes, or zucchini noodles.
- Prepare snacks like carrot and celery sticks with a side of hummus, or enjoy a small handful of almonds.

Example Recipe Idea:

Lunch could be a protein bowl with grilled chicken, roasted sweet potato cubes, steamed broccoli, and a drizzle of tahini dressing.

Pro Tip: If you're craving carbs, experiment with whole-grain options like brown rice or sprouted grain bread. These digest more slowly and provide sustained energy.

Day 3: Add Anti-Inflammatory Spices

Spices like turmeric, ginger, and cinnamon aren't just flavorful—they offer powerful anti-inflammatory properties. Incorporating these spices into your meals amplifies healing and adds depth to your dishes.

Action Steps:

- Sprinkle cinnamon onto your morning oatmeal or add ginger to your smoothie for a spicy zing.
- Use turmeric in savory meals, such as curries, soups, or marinades.

Example Recipe Idea:

Whip up a golden turmeric latte with unsweetened almond milk, a teaspoon of turmeric powder, a pinch of cinnamon, and a drizzle of honey. Or try a ginger-carrot soup as a comforting dinner option.

Pro Tip: Blend turmeric with black pepper whenever possible to boost its absorption.

Day 4: Avoid Processed Snacks

Processed snacks like chips, candy, and packaged granola bars often contain hidden sugars and unhealthy fats that hinder your progress. Swap these for whole food snacks that nourish your body.

Action Steps:

- Stock your fridge with easy-to-grab options like apple slices with almond butter, hard-boiled eggs, or a small mix of raw nuts and seeds.
- Avoid impulsive takeout by preparing simple meals at home, using leftovers from previous dinners for ease.

Example Recipe Idea:

For a mid-afternoon snack, slice up a cucumber and dip it in guacamole or hummus. Pair with a handful of baby carrots for a crunchy, satisfying option.

Pro Tip: Make a habit of checking food labels when grocery shopping. Avoid anything with long ingredient lists or names you can't pronounce.

Day 5: Focus on Lean Protein

Protein is not only essential for muscle repair and growth, but it also keeps you feeling full longer, preventing mindless snacking. The key is choosing clean, lean sources without added sugars or fats.

Action Steps:

- Build every meal around a protein source like grilled chicken, baked salmon, lightly sautéed tofu, or scrambled eggs.
- Avoid fatty cuts of red meat or processed meats like bacon or sausages, which can contribute to inflammation.

Example Recipe Idea:

Dinner could be oven-baked salmon seasoned with garlic and dill, served with roasted asparagus and a quinoa side salad.

Pro Tip: Prep proteins in bulk at the beginning of the week. For example, bake a batch of chicken breasts, or cook a pot of lentils to store for easy use in salads and soups.

Day 6: Increase Vegetables

Non-starchy vegetables are packed with the fiber, vitamins, and minerals your body needs to thrive. Make them the centerpiece of your meals, filling at least half of your plate.

Action Steps:

- Choose a wide variety of vegetables to keep things exciting. Aim for different colors to get the widest range of nutrients.

- Try roasting vegetables like broccoli, zucchini, cauliflower, or bell peppers with olive oil, salt, and your favorite seasonings for a delicious and easy side.

Example Recipe Idea:

For lunch, create a vibrant salad with mixed greens, cucumber, shredded carrots, roasted chickpeas, and a light vinaigrette. Add grilled chicken for a protein boost.

Pro Tip: Keep precut or frozen vegetables on hand to save time while still reaping the nutritional benefits.

Day 7: Plan Ahead

Use Day 7 to set yourself up for success in Week 2. Taking time to meal prep and plan will help you stay on track, even during busy days.

Action Steps:

- Roast a batch of mixed vegetables, grill or bake proteins, and cook simple soups or stews that you can store for the week ahead.
- Portion out meals into containers so you can grab them as needed.

Example Recipe Idea:

Make a big pot of chicken and vegetable soup, portioning it into individual containers for reheating throughout the week. Pair it with a side of dark leafy greens to round out the meal.

Pro Tip: Write down your Week 2 meal ideas and grocery list ahead of grocery shopping day. Having a plan makes sticking to the RAD Diet easier and less stressful.

By the end of Week 1, you'll likely notice a decrease in bloating and swelling. You'll have more energy and feel good knowing you've removed common dietary triggers. This week is only the beginning—use what you've learned as a stepping stone for the next two weeks. You're building a strong foundation for lasting change, one meal at a time. Stick with it—you're doing great!

Week 2: Nourish & Replenish

Now it's time to nourish your body back to health and give it the essential nutrients it needs. Week 2 is all about adding variety, focusing on foods that support your lymphatic system, and replenishing your energy levels with nutrient-dense, whole foods.

This week introduces key nutrients that play a role in improving circulation, fighting inflammation, and providing lasting energy. You'll focus on creating a well-rounded diet that sustains the progress you made while keeping the meals exciting and satisfying.

Goals for Week 2:

- *Add Variety*: Incorporate colorful fruits and vegetables to maximize your nutrient intake.

- ***Prioritize Lymphatic Support***: Introduce water-rich and collagen-boosting foods for better lymphatic flow and skin health.
- ***Stay Consistent with Clean Eating***: Build on Week 1's progress by sticking to anti-inflammatory choices.

This week will help you feel energized, light, and more in tune with what your body needs.

Daily Breakdown for Week 2:

Day 8: Bring in Omega-3s

Omega-3 fatty acids are known for their powerful anti-inflammatory properties, making them a critical addition to your diet. These healthy fats help reduce swelling, support brain function, and improve overall cell health.

Action Steps:

- Include 1-2 servings of omega-3-rich foods in your meals. Good options are fatty fish like salmon, mackerel, or sardines, as well as plant-based alternatives like chia seeds, ground flaxseeds, or walnuts.
- Add flavor to your meals with fresh herbs and spices. For instance, rub salmon with a mix of olive oil, garlic, and lemon juice before baking or grilling.

Example: Make a simple salmon recipe by baking a fillet seasoned with lemon, dill, and a little olive oil. Pair it with roasted asparagus and a scoop of quinoa for a complete meal.

Pro Tip: If you're not a fan of fish, try adding a teaspoon of ground flaxseed to your morning oatmeal or blending it into a smoothie for similar benefits.

Day 9: Add Magnesium-Rich Foods

Magnesium is essential for muscle relaxation, energy production, and reducing bloating—common concerns with lipedema. Incorporating magnesium-rich foods is a simple way to boost this nutrient daily.

Action Steps:

- Add leafy greens like spinach or kale to at least one meal. These greens are magnesium powerhouses.
- Snack on nuts and seeds like almonds, pumpkin seeds, or sunflower seeds. A small handful can go a long way in replenishing your magnesium levels.

Example: Toss together a leafy green salad with spinach, walnuts, sliced strawberries, and a drizzle of olive oil. Pair it with a boiled egg or grilled chicken for protein.

Pro Tip: If you're making a stir-fry or soup, toss in an extra handful of cooked spinach or kale. It blends in seamlessly while increasing the nutrient content of your dish.

Day 10: Focus on Vitamin C

Vitamin C doesn't just help your immune system—it promotes collagen production, which is crucial for skin elasticity and repair. This nutrient also helps strengthen connective tissues, which can benefit those managing lipedema.

Action Steps:

- Add a serving of citrus fruits, such as oranges, grapefruits, or mandarins, to your snacks or breakfast.
- Use fresh lemon juice to enhance the flavor of salads, grilled proteins, or cooked vegetables.

Example: Start your day with a refreshing smoothie made from 1 cup of spinach, half a frozen banana, a handful of mixed berries, and the juice of half an orange. Blend with water or unsweetened almond milk.

Pro Tip: Red bell peppers are another excellent source of vitamin C. Slice them up and pair them with hummus or add them to your stir-fry.

Day 11: Stay Hydrated with Lymph-Support Foods

Hydration is essential for improving lymphatic drainage. This is the perfect day to focus on water-rich vegetables and fruits, which not only hydrate your body but also contribute vital nutrients.

Action Steps:

- Add cucumbers, celery, watermelon, and herbs like parsley to your meals to boost hydration.
- Make an herbal tea or infused water with cucumber slices, fresh mint, and lemon. Drink this throughout the day to increase your water intake.

Example: Create a light, hydrating soup with zucchini, celery, carrots, parsley, and chicken broth. Add shredded chicken or tofu for a protein boost.

Pro Tip: Snack on crunchy, water-rich vegetables like celery sticks or cucumber slices when you need something light and refreshing.

Day 12: Rotate Protein Sources

Variety is important when it comes to protein. This day encourages you to explore the many clean, lean protein options available to you. Mixing things up keeps your diet interesting and ensures you're getting a diverse range of nutrients.

Action Steps:

- If you had mostly poultry last week, try integrating fish, eggs, or plant-based proteins like lentils and chickpeas.
- Aim to include protein in every meal to support muscle health and stabilize blood sugar.

Example: Make a warm lentil and vegetable bowl with roasted brussels sprouts, cherry tomatoes, and a tahini drizzle. Add a soft-boiled egg on top for extra protein.

Pro Tip: Prep a variety of protein-rich ingredients at the start of the week (e.g., boil eggs, roast chicken, or cook a pot of lentils) so they're easy to add to meals.

Day 13: Balance Your Plate

Learn to create balanced plates that include all the macronutrients your body needs—protein, healthy fats, and fiber-rich carbs.

Action Steps:

- Use the "plate method" where half of your plate is vegetables, a quarter is lean protein, and the other quarter is a whole grain or starchy vegetable.
- Add a small serving of healthy fat, such as avocado slices, olive oil, or a tablespoon of nuts.

Example: For dinner, try grilled chicken with steamed broccoli, roasted sweet potato wedges, and a drizzle of olive oil.

Pro Tip: Keep healthy oils like olive or avocado oil on hand to easily add good fats to your meals. Avoid seed oils or overly processed versions.

Day 14: Try New Recipes

Keep things exciting by exploring new recipes that fit the RAD Diet principles. Experimenting with flavors and ingredients helps ensure you enjoy the process and stay consistent.

Action Steps:

- Pick one or two new recipes to try this week and add the ingredients to your shopping list.
- Opt for recipes highlighting seasonal ingredients for maximum flavor and nutritional value.

Example: Make zucchini noodles with grass-fed turkey meatballs and a sugar-free marinara sauce. Sprinkle with fresh basil and grated parmesan.

Pro Tip: Bookmark or save your favorite new recipes so you can rotate them into your regular meal plan.

By the end of Week 2, you'll feel more energized and well-nourished, with a deeper understanding of how food can support your body. You'll also build confidence in preparing meals that help with inflammation and lymphatic health. Keep this momentum going as you move into Week 3, where you'll learn to sustain these changes long-term.

Week 3: Long-Term Sustainability

You've made it to Week 3, and now it's time to turn all that progress into lasting habits. This final week is about fine-tuning your approach and building a routine based on consistency and flexibility. The RAD Diet doesn't require perfection—it's about making thoughtful choices that work for you while still maintaining the principles that reduce inflammation and support your lymphatic health.

Goals for Week 3:

- *Maintain Balance*: Keep including anti-inflammatory foods like vegetables, lean proteins, and healthy fats in your meals while avoiding the major triggers you identified in the earlier weeks.
- *Create Routines*: Incorporate meal prep, balanced portions, and hydration into your weekly schedule.
- *Practice Flexibility*: Allow yourself occasional indulgences while staying mindful of how different foods make your body feel.

You've built a strong foundation in the first two weeks. Now, you'll focus on solidifying these habits in a way that fits into your lifestyle for the long term.

Daily Breakdown for Week 3:

Day 15: Stick with What Works

You likely have some favorite meals by now—recipes you enjoyed making and felt great eating. Use those as the base for your week.

Action Steps:

- Choose 2 or 3 go-to breakfasts, lunches, and dinners from Weeks 1 and 2.
- Make a shopping list with these meals in mind and include enough ingredients to cover your week.
- Lean into routines by preparing a few staple items in advance (e.g., chopping vegetables or batch-cooking grains like quinoa).

Example: If you loved the grilled salmon with roasted veggies from Week 2, double or triple the recipe this time and portion leftovers into containers for a quick lunch or dinner.

Pro Tip: Repeating meals doesn't mean things have to be boring. Use different herbs, spices, or cooking methods to maintain variety. For instance, try baking or air-frying fish instead of grilling, or swapping roasted broccoli with sautéed asparagus.

Day 16: Focus on Moderation

Cravings for treats might come up this week—and that's okay. Instead of going cold turkey, practice moderation by fitting small indulgences into your plan without guilt.

Action Steps:

- Take a mindful approach to treats. Enjoy them slowly and notice how they taste.
- Keep a healthier version of your preferred snack on hand. For example, opt for a square or two of dark chocolate (70% or more cocoa) instead of milk chocolate.

Example: If you're craving something sweet, make a smoothie bowl with frozen berries, a splash of almond milk, and just a pinch of honey or stevia for sweetness. Add some unsweetened shredded coconut or a few walnuts on top for texture.

Pro Tip: Limit portion sizes for indulgences to single servings. This makes it easier to enjoy without falling off track.

Remember, moderation isn't cheating; it's about finding balance and feeling satisfied so you can stay consistent over time.

Day 17: Keep Moving

The RAD Diet works even better when paired with gentle exercise that improves circulation and helps lymphatic drainage. Incorporating movement into your daily routine can make a big difference.

Action Steps:

- Choose an activity that feels good to your body—walking, yoga, Pilates, stretching, swimming, or low-impact strength exercises.
- Schedule 20-30 minutes of movement into your day. For example, take a brisk walk after lunch or do a short yoga session in the morning.

Example: Try a lymphatic-friendly yoga routine that focuses on gentle stretches and deep breathing. Poses like legs up-the-wall, child's pose, or twists can encourage circulation.

Pro Tip: If fitting exercise into your busy schedule feels overwhelming, start by carving out 5 minutes. Even a little bit of movement is better than none, and it can build momentum for longer sessions.

Combine this physical activity with meals that fuel your body. Aim for balanced plates with proteins, fats, and fibrous carbs to keep your energy steady.

Day 18: Cook in Batches

On busy days, having ready-made meals will keep you from reaching for less healthy, processed options. Batch cooking makes sticking to the RAD Diet easier and reduces stress during the week.

Action Steps:

- Dedicate 1-2 hours to prepare meals for the next few days. Focus on simple recipes that can be doubled or tripled.
- Make versatile staples like grilled chicken, roasted vegetables, quinoa, or soups that work across multiple meals.

Example: Cook a big pot of lentil soup or roasted vegetable quinoa salad. Store the leftovers in individual containers so they're ready to grab for lunch or dinner throughout the week.

Pro Tip: If you get bored easily, use batch-cooked staples as a base and mix things up with toppings or sauces. For instance, use roasted sweet potatoes as a side one day and the base for a veggie-packed bowl the next.

Batch cooking is a lifesaver not just for Week 3 but for the long term as well. It sets you up for success when life gets busy.

Day 19: Check Your Progress

Take time to reflect on how you've felt over the past few weeks. Tracking your progress keeps you motivated and helps you identify what's working and where you might need to adjust.

Action Steps:

- Write down your observations. How are your energy levels, mood, swelling, or discomfort compared to Day 1?
- If you've noticed a particular food or routine made a big difference, highlight that and make it a priority.
- If there are areas you're struggling with, note those too, and brainstorm simple changes to improve.

Example: If eliminating processed foods reduces bloating, but you're finding it hard to give up your favorite chips, consider making a homemade alternative like baked zucchini chips with sea salt.

Pro Tip: Use a journal or a phone app to track progress over time. Celebrate the wins, no matter how small.

Taking time to reflect will show you how far you've come and keep you focused on your goals.

Day 20: Avoid Perfectionism

Eating well isn't about being perfect. It's about making smart, consistent choices most of the time and being kind to yourself when things don't go as planned.

Action Steps:

- Avoid overly strict rules that feel discouraging in the long term.

- If you have an off day, get back on track at the next meal. Don't dwell on slip-ups—they don't undo all your progress.

Example: If you had a burger and fries at a social event, follow it up with a nutrient-rich meal like a colorful veggie quinoa salad or turkey and avocado lettuce wraps. Balance is key.

Pro Tip: Focus on progress, not perfection. Over time, these small, consistent efforts add up.

Remember, life happens, and there's room for flexibility while still staying committed to the RAD Diet.

Day 21: Celebrate Your Success

Now it's time to celebrate your hard work and set yourself up for continued success.

Action Steps:

- Reflect on everything you learned over the past three weeks.
- What are one or two habits you feel confident carrying forward? Focus on those first.
- Treat yourself—whether it's making a favorite RAD-friendly meal, enjoying a spa day, or simply taking a relaxing break.

Example: Plan a self-care day filled with activities you enjoy. For instance, take a calming bath, read your favorite book with a cup of herbal tea, or get outside for a peaceful walk in nature.

Pro Tip: Write a simple meal plan for the next week to maintain your momentum, and keep experimenting with recipes to stay excited about the RAD Diet.

By the end of Week 3, you'll have a personalized approach to the RAD Diet, allowing you to maintain these habits effortlessly. You've set the stage for better health, lower inflammation, and a sustainable way to manage lipedema through nutrition.

Lifestyle Habits to Support Lipedema Management

Managing lipedema isn't just about what you eat. Your lifestyle plays a big role in improving your symptoms and supporting overall health. From gentle movement to stress management, self-care, and supplements, small daily habits can make a significant difference in how you feel. This chapter focuses on practical, approachable strategies to help you integrate these habits alongside the RAD Diet.

The Role of Movement: Gentle Exercises to Improve Circulation

Exercise can feel tricky when dealing with lipedema, especially if you experience pain or discomfort. The good news is that movement doesn't have to be high-intensity to help. Gentle exercises improve circulation, support lymphatic drainage, and can relieve tightness or swelling.

Types of Gentle Exercises to Try:

- *Walking*: A simple, low-impact way to encourage circulation. Start with short walks around your

neighborhood, gradually increasing time or distance at your own pace.
- ***Swimming or Aqua Aerobics***: The buoyancy of water reduces pressure on your joints while helping improve circulation. Aqua therapy is especially helpful for those experiencing pain or heaviness in their legs.
- ***Yoga or Pilates***: Both focus on slow, deliberate movements that strengthen muscles, improve flexibility, and gently promote circulation. Look for beginner or restorative yoga routines that emphasize relaxation.
- ***Stationary Biking or Elliptical***: These cardio options are easy on the joints and allow you to maintain a steady, controlled pace.

Tips for Staying Active:

- Wear compression garments during exercise to support your lymphatic system and reduce discomfort.
- Focus on consistency rather than intensity. Aim for 15–30 minutes of activity at least three to five days a week.
- Listen to your body—if you feel pain or fatigue, take a break.

Regular movement doesn't just benefit your body; it can also be a mood booster. Find an activity you enjoy, and remember that any movement counts.

Managing Stress & Reducing Inflammation Holistically

Stress has a powerful effect on the body and can worsen inflammation, making symptoms of lipedema harder to manage. Finding ways to reduce and manage stress is just as important as eating well or exercising.

Practical Stress-Reduction Techniques:

1. *Mindfulness or Meditation*: Set aside five minutes a day to focus on deep breathing or guided meditation. Apps like Calm or Headspace can get you started.
2. *Gentle Stretching*: Spend a few minutes stretching in the morning or evening to release tension.
3. *Spend Time Outside*: Even a short walk in nature or sitting in the sun can improve your mood and help lower stress.
4. *Practice Gratitude*: Write down three things you're grateful for each day to shift your focus to positivity.

Reducing Exposure to Everyday Stressors:

- Limit time spent on social media or watching the news if it leaves you feeling overwhelmed.
- Organize your space to reduce visual clutter and create a calming environment.
- Set boundaries, especially with work or relationships, to protect your time and energy.

Stress can't be eliminated entirely, but building healthy habits to manage it can reduce its impact on your body over time.

Sleep, Recovery, and Self-Care Practices for Lipedema

Sleep and recovery are essential for managing inflammation and promoting healing. Poor sleep can raise cortisol levels, a stress hormone that can worsen inflammation. Prioritizing rest and self-care helps your body repair itself and function better overall.

Improving Your Sleep Quality:

- *Stick to a Consistent Schedule*: Go to bed and wake up at the same time every day, even on weekends.
- *Create a Relaxing Bedtime Routine*: Dim the lights, avoid screens for an hour before bed, and consider calming activities like reading, light stretching, or taking a warm bath.
- *Sleep Environment*: Invest in a comfortable mattress, supportive pillows, and blackout curtains to create a quiet, dark, and cool sleeping space.

If falling asleep is difficult, try progressive muscle relaxation—start by tensing and releasing your toes, then gradually work up your body.

Self-Care Practices to Support Your Body:

- ***Lymphatic Massage***: Stimulating the lymphatic system through gentle massage can ease swelling and improve drainage. A physical therapist or specialist can teach you the proper techniques to use at home.
- ***Epsom Salt Baths***: Taking a warm bath with Epsom salts can help relax muscles and reduce inflammation.
- ***Skin Care***: Keep your skin moisturized and check for any signs of irritation, as lipedema can make the skin more sensitive. Use fragrance-free lotions or oils, and avoid harsh soaps.

Recovery isn't just about rest; it's about listening to your body and giving it what it needs to heal. Prioritize taking moments for yourself and building a routine that replenishes your energy.

Supplements: Do You Need Them?

Supplements aren't a cure for lipedema, but certain ones may help support your lymphatic system and decrease inflammation when combined with the RAD Diet.

Consider These Supplements:

1. ***Omega-3 Fatty Acids***: Found in fish oil, omega-3s are known for their anti-inflammatory benefits. If you're not eating fatty fish regularly, a high-quality omega-3 supplement might support your diet.

2. ***Vitamin D***: Many people are deficient in vitamin D, which plays a role in immune health and reduces inflammation. Speak with your doctor about getting your levels checked.
3. ***Magnesium***: Known for its muscle-relaxing properties, magnesium can help manage cramping or tension. It's available in supplement form or as an Epsom salt for soaking in baths.
4. ***Curcumin (Turmeric Extract)***: Curcumin, the active compound in turmeric, has proven anti-inflammatory properties. Consider taking a supplement with black pepper extract to improve absorption.

Tips for Using Supplements Safely:

- Talk to your doctor before adding any new supplements, especially if you're on medication.
- Focus on food first—supplements are meant to fill in gaps, not replace a balanced diet.
- Follow dosage instructions carefully. Taking more than recommended won't speed up results and could potentially cause harm.

Supplements can provide added support, but they're most effective when combined with good nutrition and healthy habits.

Lifestyle habits are powerful tools for managing lipedema. Gentle movement improves circulation, stress-reduction techniques promote calm and ease inflammation, quality sleep supports recovery, and targeted self-care helps you feel your best.

How to Maintain the RAD Diet Long-Term

The key to success with the RAD Diet lies in consistency, flexibility, and finding balance over time. Here's how to make it a lasting part of your lifestyle:

1. ***Keep Things Simple***: Stick to the basics of the RAD Diet with anti-inflammatory, nutrient-dense meals. Gradually explore new recipes, rotate your favorites, and prep staples like veggies, proteins, and grains to save time and reduce stress.
2. ***Adjust for Your Lifestyle***: The RAD Diet is flexible for busy schedules, focusing on whole foods, hydration, and nutrient balance. When dining out, opt for simple meals like grilled proteins and veggies, and keep healthy frozen options at home for convenience.
3. ***Practice Progress, Not Perfection***: It's okay to stray from your diet occasionally. Focus on your next meal and return to healthy habits. The goal is consistency, not perfection.
4. ***Revisit Your WHY***: Stay motivated on the RAD Diet by reminding yourself of your "why," whether it's reducing inflammation, boosting energy, or managing lipedema.

Sticking to the RAD Diet long-term is all about balance, flexibility, and keeping your goals in mind. By making small, consistent efforts, you can turn healthy eating into a sustainable lifestyle.

Common Pitfalls & How to Overcome Them

Lipedema management can feel overwhelming at times, particularly when building new habits. Here are some common challenges readers face and tips to help you avoid or overcome them:

1. ***Feeling Discouraged by Slow Progress***: Managing lipedema takes time, and results can sometimes feel slow. Remember, the small changes you're making add up over months and years. Celebrate non-scale victories like reduced swelling, higher energy levels, or simply feeling more in tune with your body.
2. ***Social Events & Peer Pressure***: Events like parties, gatherings, or eating out can feel stressful when trying to stick to the RAD Diet. Plan ahead by eating a light, healthy meal beforehand, looking at menus online, or bringing a dish you know aligns with your goals. If someone questions your choices, focus on what makes you feel good rather than explaining your diet in detail.
3. ***Temptation to Fall Back on Old Habits***: It's normal to have cravings during stressful times. Satisfy them in moderation by choosing healthier alternatives, like

air-popped popcorn or dark chocolate, instead of overly processed options. Focus on balance, not restriction.

4. **Feeling Isolated**: Having support, like an accountability partner or community, is key to successfully adapting to the RAD Diet and avoiding feelings of isolation.

Managing lipedema comes with challenges, but small, consistent changes and the right strategies can make a big difference over time. Remember, progress is a journey—celebrate every step forward and lean on support when you need it.

Additional Resources & Support Groups

You don't need to do this alone. There are many resources and communities available to support you on your lipedema and RAD Diet journey. Here are suggestions to help you stay connected and informed:

1. **Books, Blogs, and Social Media**: Explore books and blogs that focus on anti-inflammatory eating, lymphatic health, or lipedema management. Instagram, Facebook, and YouTube often have communities where people share meal ideas, success stories, and challenges. Just be sure to choose content that resonates with you and keeps a positive tone.

2. ***Support Groups***: Consider joining a support group for people managing lipedema or similar conditions. Look for groups through local hospitals, community centers, or online forums. These groups can provide empathy, advice, and ongoing encouragement from people who truly understand your experience.
3. ***Professional Support***: Working with a healthcare provider, nutritionist, or physical therapist can be invaluable, especially when you're feeling stuck or need personalized guidance. These professionals can help you adapt the RAD Diet to suit your unique needs and goals.
4. ***RAD Diet Resources***: Keep using your guide as a resource! Revisit chapters when you're looking for meal inspiration, need motivation to move, or want to refine your habits. You've already got a solid foundation to work from.

Remember, you're not alone on this journey—support and resources are always within reach. Stay connected, seek guidance when needed, and keep building on the progress you've already made!

Conclusion

Thank you for taking the time to explore the RAD Diet Guide. Reaching this point shows your dedication to understanding and managing lipedema, and that commitment matters. Every piece of knowledge gained here empowers you to make informed choices that suit your unique needs.

Managing lipedema can feel overwhelming, but small, consistent changes lead to noticeable progress. Each step—whether it's swapping out inflammatory foods, squeezing in gentle movement, or prioritizing self-care—builds a stronger foundation for symptom relief and better health. It's not about striving for perfection but about making choices that work for you and your body one day at a time.

The RAD Diet supports your body, not through restriction but by fueling it with what it needs to function its best. Choosing anti-inflammatory, nutrient-dense foods while avoiding common triggers helps reduce tenderness, ease swelling, and support better energy levels. Pairing these habits with gentle exercise and self-care ensures your approach stays balanced and sustainable.

If you face challenges, remember that progress is a process. Be patient with yourself. The small victories—less swelling, improved mobility, or even just feeling more at ease—should be celebrated. You're creating a lifestyle that supports your well-being and helps you feel in control.

Above all, don't forget to give yourself credit for your effort. You've taken an important step by completing this guide, and with each meal, movement, and mindful moment, you get closer to your health goals. Stay consistent, stay hopeful, and stay kind to yourself along the way.

FAQs

What is the RAD Diet, and who is it for?

The RAD Diet, or Rare Adipose Diet, is designed specifically for managing lipedema. It focuses on reducing inflammation, improving lymphatic health, and stabilizing blood sugar through nutrient-dense, anti-inflammatory foods. It's tailored for anyone living with lipedema who seeks practical and sustainable dietary changes to manage symptoms.

How does the RAD Diet help with lipedema symptoms?

The RAD Diet emphasizes anti-inflammatory foods, such as leafy greens and omega-3-rich sources, while reducing pro-inflammatory triggers like refined sugars and processed foods. This approach helps reduce swelling, improve circulation, and balance blood sugar, which can positively affect pain and mobility.

Is the RAD Diet only for weight loss?

No, the RAD Diet isn't primarily about weight loss. It focuses on healing and managing lipedema symptoms by targeting inflammation, boosting lymphatic health, and improving metabolic function, rather than solely aiming for calorie reduction.

How does the RAD Diet differ from regular diets?

Unlike many traditional weight-loss diets, the RAD Diet addresses the unique needs of those with lipedema. It doesn't prioritize calorie restriction or rapid weight loss. Instead, it focuses on healing the body with foods that reduce swelling, support the lymphatic system, and provide long-lasting energy.

What types of foods should I focus on in the RAD Diet?

The RAD Diet encourages anti-inflammatory foods like leafy greens, fatty fish (such as salmon), low-glycemic carbs (like sweet potatoes or quinoa), and healthy fats (such as avocado and olive oil). It avoids processed foods, refined sugars, trans fats, and high-sodium items.

Do I need special equipment or supplements for the RAD Diet?

No special equipment is required, but meal prep tools like food containers, a blender, or spiralizer can be helpful. While some supplements, such as omega-3 fatty acids or vitamin D, can support the diet, these should be used after consulting a doctor.

How soon can I expect to see results?

Progress varies from person to person, as each individual responds differently. Some may begin to notice reduced swelling and discomfort within a few weeks, while for others, it might take a couple of months to see significant changes.

Factors such as the severity of the condition, consistency in following recommendations, and overall health can all impact the timeline. The goal is to achieve lasting, sustainable improvements rather than quick, temporary fixes, so patience and persistence are key throughout the process.

References and Helpful Links

Lipedema. (2025, February 18). Cleveland Clinic. https://my.clevelandclinic.org/health/diseases/17175-lipedema

Herbst, K. L. (2012). Rare adipose disorders (RADs) masquerading as obesity. Acta Pharmacologica Sinica, 33(2), 155–172. https://doi.org/10.1038/aps.2011.153

Lipedema: symptoms, treatment, causes, and more. (n.d.). WebMD. https://www.webmd.com/women/lipedema-symptoms-treatment-causes

RAD diet for lipedema. (n.d.). https://www.therapygarments.com/rad-diet-lipedema.html?srsltid=AfmBOopzJO86YN53DfBewglS0kEiCGpazRI9IZUfdHf4X4iaH1VjQeao

RAD diet food. (n.d.). Pinterest. https://www.pinterest.com/hatten0219/rad-diet-food/

LaMantia, J. (2023, May 14). Diet for lipedema. Jean LaMantia - Registered Dietitian in Toronto, ON. https://jeanlamantia.com/diet-for-lipedema/

» Diet & Supplement recommendations and Rationale for lipedema - Lipedema. (n.d.). https://www.lipedema.net/nutritious-eating-to-reduce-lipedema.html

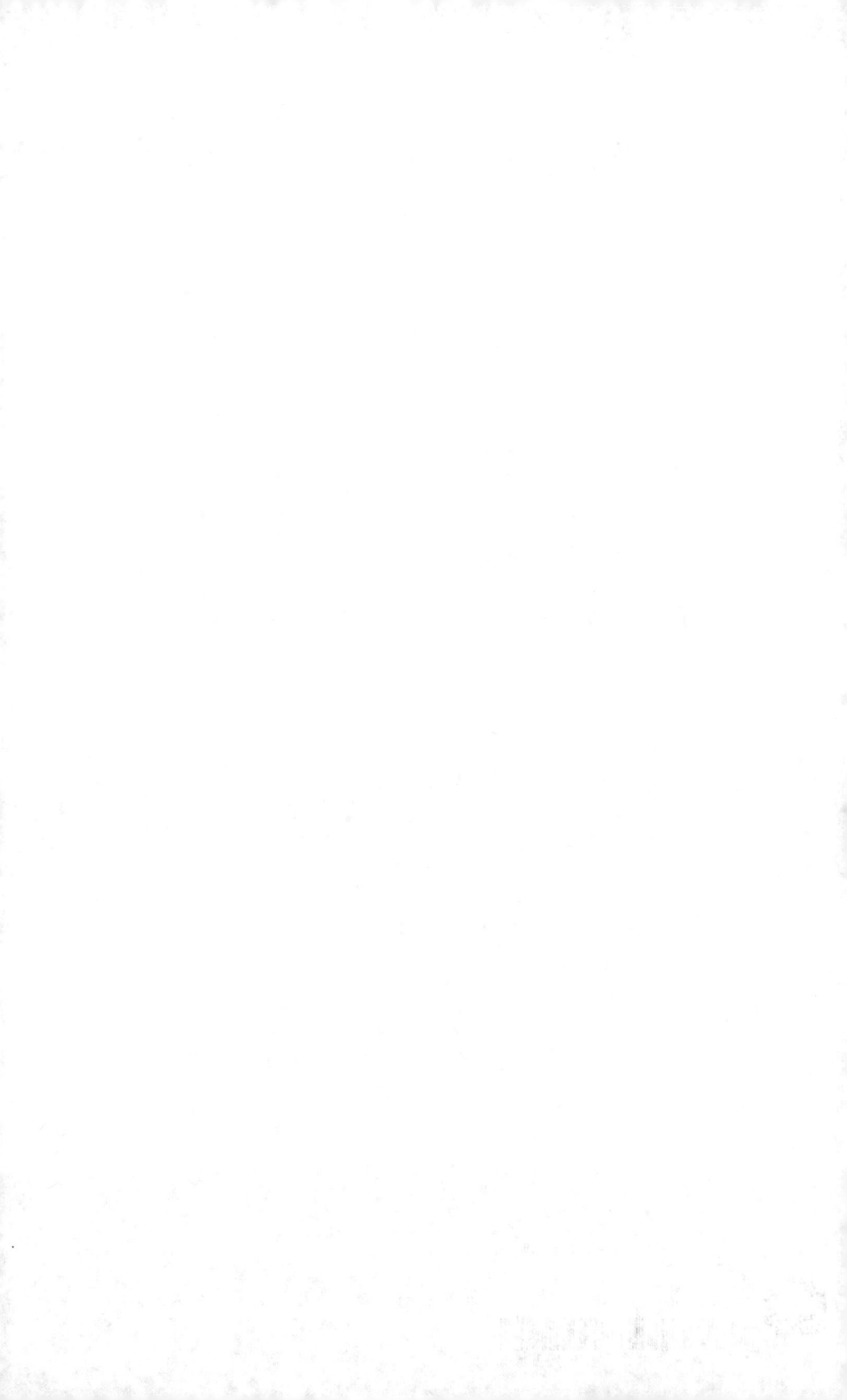

www.ingramcontent.com/pod-product-compliance
Lightning Source LLC
LaVergne TN
LVHW012029060526
838201LV00061B/4530